YOUR HIGH ENERGY LIFE

Banish Energy-Sucking Foods and Supercharge Your Days

Jadie Aranda
www.EatMyScience.com

Copyright © 2017 Jadie Aranda

All rights reserved. No part of this publication may be reproduced, distributed, or transmitted in any form or by any means, including photocopying, recording, or other electronic or mechanical methods, without the prior written permission of the publisher, except in the case of brief quotations embodied in reviews and certain other non-commercial uses permitted by copyright law.

Disclaimer

The information in this book is designed for informational purposes only. This book is not meant to be used, nor should it be used, as professional medical advice. For diagnosis or treatment of any medical problem, consult your own physician. References are provided for informational purposes only and do not constitute endorsement of any websites or other sources. The author assumes no responsibility or liability whatsoever on behalf of the purchaser or reader of the information in this book.

Contents

Dedication 2
Preface 3
Acknowledgements 5
Chapter 1 – What Could You Do with More Energy? 6
Chapter 2 – Get Your Brain in the Game 15
Chapter 3 – Processed Food 20
Chapter 4 – Sugar 34
Chapter 5 – Hydration 43
Chapter 6 – Overeating 53
Chapter 7 – Immune Response 60
Chapter 8 – Recipes for Energy 68
Conclusion 77
About the Author 78
Thank You! 79

DEDICATION

This book is dedicated to you, the reader, and your body in all its greatness. I hope this book helps you learn how to eat what your body needs, so that you have the energy to achieve your wildest dreams!

PREFACE

What are your biggest accomplishments in life?

Taking a while to come up with an answer?

What if I asked what you could accomplish if you had superhuman energy? It's easier and more fun to answer that question.

My—and probably your—excuse for not living the dream life was because I was too tired. After all the daily to-dos, I just didn't have it in me to do anything else. I started scouring the internet for The One Thing that would boost my daily energy and solve all my problems.

I should have known Google wasn't going to give me the answer. I have a degree in biology, and I know the body is more complex than a single answer that could pop up in a Google search. But I also believe that just because our bodies are complicated, that doesn't mean getting more energy has to be. We learn to use complex computers and counter-intuitive smart phones. We put a man on the moon, for goodness' sake—we should be able to learn how our bodies work best!

My research led me to write this book because I did uncover good news: you CAN have superhuman energy! In fact, you're entitled to superhuman energy—because the irony is that what I'm calling "superhuman" is simply how we are naturally designed to function as regular, ol' "human." However, we're so out of touch with how to best support a healthy human body, that we've settled for a "normal" that is severely downgraded from our natural state.

I will teach you how the way you currently eat is inhibiting your ability to live the energetic life you are meant to live. I will explain why processed foods, extra sugar, dehydration, overeating, and your unhealthy immune response to your standard diet is sucking the life right out of you. You will learn what your body truly needs to function at its highest potential, day in and day out.

Above all, you will learn that by changing what you eat, you can achieve anything you want.

Eat well, my friends. Your life depends on it.

ACKNOWLEDGEMENTS

I thought writing a book was like sailing around the world solo, isolating in the moment but with a great sense of accomplishment at the end. I was so wrong. Without these fantastic people to man the ship, I could never make the trip.

A huge thank you to:

Chandler Bolt and Self-Publishing School for breaking the creative process into logical steps for those of us who need a guide;

Micah Klug, my accountability partner for meeting with me every Wednesday to keep me on course;

Desirée Domo, my incredible editor, for polishing my thoughts and words and improving this book exponentially;

Jessica Seybold for capturing the essence of the book's message perfectly through her beautiful cover designs;

Amanda for riding the waves of emotion with me through this entire process;

My **incredible husband and two wonderful children** for reminding me why I am pursuing my passion;

and my **Mom**, for almost four decades of unconditional love, heartfelt teaching, and unparalleled support.

1
WHAT COULD YOU DO WITH MORE ENERGY?

"You only live once, but if you do it right, once is enough."

–Mae West

In this fast-paced world, our default setting is "on-the-go" and we are all more tired than ever. Many times, we go to bed regretting what we didn't accomplish during the day instead of feeling thankful for all we achieved. We just don't have the energy to do everything we need to do.

Does it take a cup of coffee, tea, or soda to get your brain going in the morning? Do you need another cup mid-morning to jumpstart your get-up-and-go? Do you fight the urge to nap after lunch?

If so, you are not alone. Daytime tiredness affects 55 to 75 percent of Americans, according to recent studies. If you search "how to get more energy" or "why do I feel tired," hundreds of articles show up in your web browser. Why?

1. People are really tired.
2. People like to write about being tired.
3. Nobody has a good answer for why we're so tired.

There are dozens of resources all over the internet on how to get more energy, but none of them truly solve the rampant tiredness that millions of people across the globe experience daily.

Until now.

This book does the solving you've been looking for. This is the blueprint for more energy in your daily life, to more productive days, to feeling like you can take on the world. It is your answer—so that you can move past the questioning and googling and live the best life you can live. Your best life requires one thing: your 100 percent. And when you're tired, 100 percent is never possible.

I've studied the human body my whole life and have a degree in Biology. I find the inner workings of this incredible machine fascinating. But like almost all of you, I didn't think about what I was eating or how it made me feel. I ate for pleasure. I ate what tasted good. I ate what was convenient.

And I fueled my body with crap.

But I didn't know it was crap. I ate what the commercials told me to eat, the only way I knew.

Then I found myself in my 30s, with two kids and a household to run and work to be done, and I was tired.

I suddenly became a coffee drinker.

I dragged myself out of bed at the last possible moment and looked forward to the weekend when I could sleep for 12 hours.

I had only enough drive to do the bare minimum at work, around the house, and for my family.

This was not the life I wanted to live. I started beating myself up about not having willpower or motivation. I went to bed feeling unproductive.

And the worst thing was that I felt like a terrible parent because there were so many things that I wanted to teach my children about life, but could only manage to throw on a video and make macaroni and cheese . . . again.

I turned to my studies in biology to examine the parts of my brain that did not seem to be working right. Where was my willpower, my excitement, my ENERGY?

One day I was deeply entrenched in reading about the brain, specifically the chemical messengers and hormones that regulate decision making—yes, I get THAT geeky when it comes to science—and I read a sentence that stopped me in my tracks:

> *"AG was also shown to interact with several other G protein-coupled receptors such as the dopamine*

receptor subtypes 1 and 2 (DRD1/2) and melanocortin receptor 3 (MC3R) in the central nervous system."[1]

Translation: Everything that happens in the brain is directly related to the food we eat.

Cue my lightbulb moment. I had read versions of that translation—i.e. "you are what you eat!"—many times before, but no such statement was ever backed up by science. Yet here it was, staring me right in the face: the scientific proof. The proof that all I needed to do was give my body the right fuel, and I could be superhuman.

When I began feeding my body (and brain!) the fuel it could actually use, my life became electrifying . . . perhaps because my very energy felt electric—like a switch had been turned on.

I started waking up feeling rested, with great ideas and inspiration flowing from the moment my eyes opened.

I was suddenly annoyingly happy toward my family, coworkers, strangers on the street, without ever feeling tired or irritable.

---

[1] François Chabot, "Interrelationships between ghrelin, insulin and glucose homeostasis: Physiological relevance," *World Journal of Diabetes* 5, no. 3 (June 15, 2014). doi:10.4239/wjd.v5.i3.328.

I was finishing projects I'd been working on without any mental glitches—no writers' block, no forgetfulness, no brain farts.

As corny as it sounds, I began accomplishing my wildest dreams. And if corny is the cost of genuine dream-catching, I welcome the label.

Right now you may be thinking a lot smaller. "If I just had more energy, I could do laundry before I run out of underwear." Fair. I get that. But having gone through it myself, I'm giving you permission to think big.

Imagine six months from now when you have the energy to go to the gym and run a 5K like you've wanted to do for years. Visualize a year from now when you decide to start your own business or become an independent contractor because you now have the energy and the drive to be more successful in your career. Or glimpse five years from now when the charity you've started and spearheaded has helped over a million people.

Whatever your dreams are, you can accomplish them, one meal at a time.

Because the lack of energy holding you back from your wildest dreams is caused by the way you eat.

It's not your fault. There are good excuses why we eat the things we eat. But rather than passively falling back on excuses, actively choose your reason to eat. The best reason is this one: to create the life you want to live. To have the freedom to accomplish whatever you want. To have the energy to live a superhuman life.

It all starts with a single meal.

But you have to start.

You have the energy to read this book right now, and you know you may not have that energy tomorrow. You owe it to yourself, to your future, to your life, to keep reading.

Do not let this book get lost in the cloud or buried under a pile of paper—unless you're equally willing to let your dreams be as easily lost or buried.

Starting your metamorphosis is as simple as turning the page or swiping a finger. All you have to do to begin maximizing your energy and upgrading your life is keep reading.

2
GET YOUR BRAIN IN THE GAME

"In order to do something you've never done, you've
got to become someone you've never been."
—Les Brown

Still reading? Color me impressed—you're on a roll, low-energy friend! Reading this book may be only the beginning of your transformation, but the good news is that you're past the hardest part: starting. Bravo.

You want the life you've never had and you're doing the thing you've never done: you're reading this book. You're on your way.

As soon as I started thinking differently, my behavior seemed to organically follow. I couldn't help being different because my mindset was different—and I was becoming the person who matched that mindset.

So let's steer your growth in the right direction. You are reading this book because you want something. What do you want? Say it out loud, right now.

Need some help getting started?

Finish this sentence: "I want more energy in my day so I can ____________."

Great! You know why you want to live a more energetic life.

Spoiler: it won't happen just by saying it. If you wake up tomorrow and eat the same breakfast and coffee and snacks and lunch and dinner, your day will not somehow be different than today.

You won't ever realize that goal if it lives only in your head. Sure, it starts there . . . but if it's going to materialize in the world, then it needs to venture beyond the confines of your imagination.

Throughout this book, I am going to give you the knowledge and the tools to feed your body better. I'm going to tell you why you should and shouldn't eat certain things so that when you have to make a decision about eating that donut in the breakroom, you know exactly what the consequences are.

I'm also going to talk about breakroom donuts a lot, because that's my weakness. If you don't have a problem with breakroom donuts, then think of your sugary nemesis every time you read "donut."

Before we dive into the nitty gritty of what you are going to eat when you want to feel superhuman, you need to get your brain in the game and commit to eating something different—after all, it's your brain that stands to benefit most.

Imagine yourself with child-like energy, punching through your day like a superhuman accomplishing all your missions. What does that version of you look like?

The you that's standing as tall as the Empire State, engaging people with smiling eyes, slashing through the items on your to do list. The you that's playing a whole game of Candyland with your toddler without wanting to chuck it out the window, whipping up a meal worthy of Gordon Ramsey's approval, watching an entire movie without falling asleep on the couch. The you that's scaling a fourteener with your best buddies, reveling in the beauty of nature, soaking in the warmth from the sun.

What does the superhuman version of yourself eat? Pizza? Soda? Donuts?

Probably not. And honestly, most of us have no idea what we should eat. Which is why we don't live superhuman lives.

Well, for you that changes today.

Your new mantra—when crafting every meal, when mulling over that donut, when passing the vending machine in the hall—is this:

When I eat better: I feel better, I think better, I live better.

Making lasting change is not an easy thing, but if you can get your brain in the game, you will be much more likely to gain the crazy superhuman energy you need to blast through your day.

3
PROCESSED FOOD

"As for butter versus margarine, I trust cows more
than chemists."

–Joan Dye Gussow

Many experts and research studies say processed foods are killing us with pesticides, chemicals, additives, artificial colors and ingredients, preservatives, and GMOs. Only a few minutes on the internet will show you that these foods are the "root of all evil."

Cool. Stop eating processed foods. That's it! Next chapter!

Just kidding. If it were that simple, companies like Nestle, Pepsico, and Kraft would not be billion-dollar enterprises. And I'm not suggesting you boycott all food manufacturers and processed foods to live your superhuman life. Because in this day and age, in our society, this would be impossible. After all, you probably want to be badass at something other than growing your own food.

But for your energy's sake, you really must limit processed foods.

So what's wrong with processed food? I'm not going to sugarcoat it. There are three main ways these foods hurt your energy levels:

1. Processed foods are missing key nutrients.
2. These foods offer low-quality energy sources.
3. Foreign particles can cause an inflammatory response.

Processed foods are missing key nutrients

Most of us have heard of the macronutrients: protein, fat, and carbohydrate. In addition to macronutrients, your body also needs a wide variety of the lesser-known micronutrients to function properly, such as vitamins, minerals, and other phytochemicals (some that we don't even know about yet!).

Micronutrients come from the food you eat. There are over 40 micronutrients identified that your body needs, but note that these are "identified." Scientists continue to study biology and nature and find compounds and chemicals that were previously unknown. How's that for humbling? We don't know everything there is to know yet . . . which explains why we've made such glaring mistakes in the past. Processing food is one of those mistakes. Unfortunately, processing food removes the diverse array of micronutrients that your body needs, whether we know about them or not.

Humans have been playing with their food for centuries. Making bread from yeast and wheat, fermenting grains to make alcohol, and adding heat to foods to make them edible. In the last 200 years, however, the industrial revolution stoked the desire to improve all aspects of life. Chemistry became a thriving industry. Electricity was routed to people's homes. New industries of food production and convenience foods grew.

The industrial revolution first taught us that we could take existing things and make them better through engineering and technology. We looked to engineering, technology, and science to create food that was safer, tastier, and lasted longer. However, in hindsight we're learning engineering and technology doesn't necessarily better everything.

The 20th century gave rise to the foods that we grew up on, the cornerstones of the current standard American diet. But their FDA approval doesn't overshadow the fact that processing has stripped them of their nutritious micronutrients.

Manufacturers enrich wheat flour with a few of the identified missing micronutrients, but not all the nutrients stripped from food during processing. In fact, they are not even the same micronutrients that were first removed from the wheat itself. This enrichment is a public supplementation program.

You are taking supplements without realizing it. Table salt is also supplemented. Manufacturers add iodine to the salt, not because it was removed from the salt during processing, but the government needed to find a way to add iodine to the standard diet, and they chose to supplement salt.

The main point is that processed foods are stripped of their micronutrients, but only a few are added back to the food before it reaches the shelf of your grocery store. And others are also added that never belonged there in the first place. A diet consisting of mostly processed foods is missing the vast array of micronutrients the body needs to work at peak performance.

When micronutrients are missing, your body enters conservation mode to save the micronutrients it does have. Conservation mode can lower metabolism and energy production, and make you feel less energized.

When the body attempts to digest processed foods, the food no longer resembles the nutrient panel that is found in nature. This makes digestion more difficult, requiring more energy and making you feel tired after meals.

What does "lowering metabolism" even mean?

The human body is a collection of chemicals that react in specific ways to produce everything from the heartbeat to brain waves to toe nails.

Metabolism is the term for all the chemical reactions that happen in the body. For these chemical reactions to occur, the body needs food for fuel, water to help break down and move molecules, and oxygen to use in the chemical reactions themselves. We can live just several weeks without food, a few days without water, but barely a couple minutes without oxygen.

The energy we feel (or don't feel) is our body's way of telling us how our metabolism is functioning. We cannot feel all the chemical reactions happening in the trillions of cells in the body. But we can feel when metabolism slows down, ramps up, or needs to recharge with sleep.

Metabolism happens at the cellular level. Imagine each cell is a manufacturing facility of a ginormous company. You are the CEO. It is your job to make sure the factories have the supplies they need to perform their jobs: food, water, oxygen. From there, they know what they are supposed to do. It's impossible to monitor trillions of factories at once. As CEO, you receive general signals for the condition of the company as a whole. Then you can make decisions about what to eat to keep metabolism running optimally.

Processed foods offer low-quality energy sources

Processed foods have proteins, carbohydrates, and fats to give us calories and energy. And one could argue that once these macronutrients are digested and broken down into their basic parts, the body treats them all the same. A glucose molecule is a glucose molecule, whether it comes from an apple or a cookie, right?

Unfortunately, it is not that simple. The way our bodies digest and absorb food is largely determined by the contents of the whole food that we eat, not just the basic macronutrients in the food.

In natural whole foods, nutrients are packaged with everything your body needs to digest and absorb the high-quality nutrition of the food. In processed foods, as we discussed earlier, many nutrients are stripped from the food or incorrectly added to the food, making the energy sources of those foods incomplete or erroneously structured.

Processing also can change the macronutrients in ways that they then no longer resemble the proteins, carbohydrates, and fats found in nature. A great example of this is trans fats.

By processing natural fats using a method known as hydrogenation, some of the fat molecules change their structure to what is known as trans structure—the same molecules in the same order, but arranged differently in space. Technically these molecules are still fats, but their trans arrangement gives them different physical properties which are helpful to food manufacturers (i.e. solidity at room temperature making them more stable to last longer on shelves without compromising taste).

Because of the trans arrangement, the body also treats the molecules in a different way. Studies show that consumption of trans fats causes an increase in heart disease, diabetes, and inflammation. Even more disturbing, most scientist and dieticians agree that trans fats have negative health effects and should be avoided, but manufacturers are still able to use them in the production of processed foods.

While this is just one example of how processed foods can have low quality, harmful energy sources, any food that is processed is treated differently in the body than the natural source. And since digestion and absorption of food take a lot of energy, if you are eating processed foods that require additional resources (energy) to break down, eating these foods will cause a drop in your overall energy level.

Foreign particles can cause inflammatory response

Low quality protein, carbohydrates, and fats can cause an immune response in the body like we discussed with trans fats, but extra chemicals and additives in processed foods can also cause an immune response and inflammation.

The body examines everything we eat to determine if it is useful or unnecessary. The basic building blocks of protein, carbohydrates, and fats are well known and the body can deal with them quickly. Micronutrients like vitamins and minerals are also easily recognizable and dealt with easily.

Chemicals that are not found in nature are not as easy for the body to deal with. When we eat processed foods that have these chemicals added to them, the body flags the foreign molecules and can cause an immune response just as if a foreign particle were to get trapped under your skin.

Think of a splinter. If you can't get it out quickly, the site of the splinter usually turns red and can get hot as the body tries to deal with the foreign particle. The same thing can happen in your digestive system.

When we eat chemicals that the body doesn't recognize, it increases our immune response and causes all kinds of problems. Swollen intestines cannot absorb nutrients as well as they need to, which means we are missing out on vital elements needed to produce maximum energy.

By eating processed foods, not only are you missing out on important nutrients that your body needs to function at a high level, you can't even absorb the nutrients you need for your basic energy needs. You don't have the nutrients necessary to maintain the energy you are looking for—the all day energy that makes you your best self.

Not all processed foods are created equal

What is processed food anyway? Another problem with websites that simply tell you to avoid processed foods is that they never even answer that question. I mean, that packaged lettuce is triple washed; that's a process. Does that mean I shouldn't eat it?

Here is a simple set of guidelines to determine the level of processing of a certain food:

1. Does it contain only one ingredient?

This is a whole food—the way nature intended it.

2. Does it have two or three ingredients?

These are things that were whole but mixed together in some way, like peanuts and salt to make peanut butter. Real peanut butter, not Jif with its seven (mostly) unnecessary ingredients.

3. Can you see whole foods in it?

For example, some nut bars have four or so ingredients, and you can physically see the whole nuts. These foods are processed, but less so than our next category.

4. Does every item look and taste exactly the same?

Think Twinkies here. One of the biggest reasons for the major processing and chemicals in our food is consistency.

Using these guidelines, it is simple to pick something up in the supermarket and determine the level of processing. This checklist lines up with other advice you will find—shop on the outer aisles of the store, buy things with less than five ingredients, and with ingredients you can pronounce.

It is this simple, but that doesn't mean it will be easy. Most of the foods in the last category are foods that we love. Part of the reason we love them is because they taste the same, every time. A Twinkie tastes just like a Twinkie, whether you ate it 20 years ago or today. Perhaps we crave reliability more than anything.

Next, we are going to discuss sugar. If processed food is the root of all evil, then sugar is the flower of all evil. The beautiful, addictive flower.

4
SUGAR

"Sweetness is not in itself unhealthy, we simply eat
only the most unhealthy kind of sweetness."
—Giulia Enders

Carbohydrates, which are the macronutrient made up of sugars, are an integral part of what we eat. You will see that carbohydrates are the basic energy source for all cells. We need sugar to survive; glucose is the body and brain's main source of energy.

So does that mean that more sugar gives you more energy? Unfortunately, no. Too much sugar overwhelms your system and causes you to crash.

Carbohydrates from any source are basically used in the body in the same way. It is the amount absorbed at any given time that causes variation in the body's response to the carbohydrates. The carbohydrates we consume are digested differently and at different rates. Not all carbs are created equal.

For most healthy young people, this crash in energy

feels more like a dip, and it is an indication to grab another cup of coffee or a sugary snack. Eventually, this dip becomes more and more noticeable until you start feeling very tired most of the day.

I suspect many of you reading this book have exactly this problem. What makes it even more difficult is that we do not know we are hurting our bodies until the damage is so severe we have to take drastic measures. If your energy dips throughout the day become more of a constant low energy state, then it's time to change your diet.

Let's face it: you're not as young as you used to be. When we were younger, we could eat all the candy, ice cream, milk shakes, cake, SUGAR that we wanted—and the worst consequence that ever happened was a tummy ache.

Now that you are in your 30s or beyond, you ask for a small piece of birthday cake. You start buying individually wrapped candies instead of gallons of ice cream. That donut from the breakroom tastes soooo good—but a little while later, you're sitting at your desk and can't remember what you are supposed to be working on. Can't you just take a nap first, then work?

What is happening here? Isn't sugar supposed to be the body's main fuel source? Shouldn't it give you energy? Why don't you feel like running around the backyard for four hours after a glass of chocolate milk like a five-year-old?

The body uses sugar for fuel. Simple sugars from processed foods and desserts are a quick, powerful source of fuel—though not necessarily the best quality for the body. They are so powerful, eating them is like adding jet fuel to your car. It is more fuel than your body needs.

As kids, our bodies use energy rapidly because we are growing quickly, constantly learning new things (yes, the brain uses a lot of energy!), and we also naturally eat exactly as much as our bodies can use and then stop. Even for kids, however, simple sugars are like jet fuel.

As adults, we don't need as much energy. We stop growing, and our needs become dependent on how active we are. We also don't have time to run around in the backyard for an hour after we eat that donut.

The biggest impact on the body is when that jet fuel hits your bloodstream, which happens extremely quickly when you eat a sugary snack or soda. The release of insulin by the pancreas happens as a direct result of your blood sugar level. If you eat simple, processed sugars, your blood sugar is going to get really high, really fast, which is going to cause your pancreas to release a lot of insulin really fast.

Too much, too fast, in fact.

Our bodies are designed to digest whole, natural foods. Foods that are high in simple sugars don't exist very often in nature. And even when they do, they are contained in a rich complex of other fibers and nutrients, and do not impact blood sugar the same way that processed sugars do.

The body is expecting complex sugars and expects that an influx of sugars will be followed by more, and insulin levels remain elevated after the blood sugar is lowered. If a high amount of insulin is released in response to a high blood sugar, it will take insulin levels longer to come down. While the high level of insulin is finally coming down, it still signals to the cells to take sugar out of the blood. This results in a condition known as hypoglycemia, or low blood sugar.

At this point, your cells are like, "OK, hello? Where's our fuel?"

Your body requires a relatively stable amount of blood sugar to function properly, so when your blood sugar goes too low, you feel tired, and crash.

How to avoid the sugar crash

The key to avoiding the draining sugar crash is to make sure the blood sugar/insulin spike cycle doesn't occur. How do you do that?

1. Don't eat sweets on an empty stomach.

Eating dessert after a meal usually doesn't cause a sugar crash. Why? Because our bodies are busy digesting complex proteins, fats, and carbohydrates. The sugar takes longer to get into the bloodstream and enters more slowly, so there is no insulin spike. If you are going to have sugar, do it after you've eaten something nutritious.

2. Don't eat sugar by itself.

OK, no one's spooning the white stuff directly into their mouths. But you can choose to eat sweets in combination with more nutritious foods. For example, nuts are an excellent source of fat and protein. Eat some whole nuts with chocolate, à la chocolate peanut clusters or bars with whole nuts like a Kind bar. Fruits have a lot of sugar too, but they come in a high fiber package. These sweet snacks have less of an impact on blood sugar so you can enjoy a sugary treat but avoid the sugar crash.

3. Know which sweets have the most and least sugar.

Chocolate is the quintessential sugary treat, but not all chocolate is created equal. Dark chocolate has way less sugar than milk chocolate, and different brands add different amounts of sugar based on the desired flavor outcome and the process they use. No matter what your weakness is—be it chocolate, ice cream, or gum drops, do a little research to find treats that will satisfy your cravings with less sugar. A simple swap can save you from the sugar crash. You can have your cake and eat it too!

4. Make sure your sugary treat has real sugar.

There are many studies on the effects of artificial sweeteners, and the results are very bad news for the body. The powerful brain will get the body ready when it knows something is coming, like when you start salivating at the thought of the chimichangas at your favorite Mexican food restaurant. When your brain senses it is getting sugar from something sweet, it readies the body for that influx of fuel. When there is no fuel because you consumed some other chemical that just tasted sweet, it can have negative effects on your blood sugar regulation.

5. Never drink your sugar.

Sugary drinks such as soda have no nutritional value at all. A bunch of sugar in liquid form will go right to your blood and initiate the insulin/blood sugar cycle faster than you can say "liter-a-cola" . . . Super Troopers style.

Sugary drinks—particularly soda—give a triple whammy. Not only do they cause blood sugar issues, they are also full of unnatural chemicals that can cause an immune response and keeps you from what you truly should be drinking much more of: water. The elixir of life is the subject of our next chapter.

It is true that if we got rid of all the sugary treats and drinks in the world, we would be a healthier human population for it. But the fact is we like sugary stuff.

Nobody would be making it if we weren't buying it. What we're missing is this: despite the seeming lack of possibilities, it is possible to enjoy sugar responsibly.

5
HYDRATION

"Water is life, and clean water means health."
                                    –Audrey Hepburn

What we drink is the easiest habit to change. It also has the biggest impact on your energy level. This is because most of us drink crap that depletes us instead of drinking water that nourishes us.

As it relates to energy, water provides three extremely important functions. The most important function of water is in the chemical reaction of ATP, the energy currency of the cells. But first, we need to understand what ATP is!

What is ATP?

Metabolism in every cell runs on the same energy source: adenosine triphosphate, or ATP. ATP is often called the energy "currency" of cell metabolism. ATP is required for all the cells' functions, whether it's flexing a muscle, making connections in the brain for memory, or fighting off infection. I know words like adenosine triphosphate are pretty sciency, and it really isn't important that you memorize how to spell it or even remember what ATP stands for. The important thing to remember is that these are the rechargeable batteries that supply your energy throughout the day. ATP is the only form of energy your cells can use.

The food we eat is broken down during digestion and absorbed in our intestines. First carbohydrates, then fats, and finally proteins if needed are sent to each cell, which uses the calories to make ATP.

Imagine ATP is the dollar in the U.S. If you have pesos, euros, or dirhams, you will need to exchange them for dollars before you can use the currency. In the same way, the body converts carbohydrates, fats, and proteins into ATP.

As a final note, the primary function of carbohydrates is to supply quick energy. Cells will always use sugar (carbohydrates) to make ATP first. If sugar is not available, fats are used to make the ATP. Fats serve several functions in the body, but the primary function is to store and supply energy when needed. Cells can use protein to make ATP, but this is a last resort. Proteins have much more important functions in the body.

ATP and water

The energy from ATP is released by adding water. If you are dehydrated, your body can't release the energy. It's like having money in the bank but forgetting your pin number on a bank holiday. The money is there, you just can't get to it. No energy.

The second critical function of water in your body is the movement of chemicals. Cells perform different functions based on the concentration of chemicals, including signaling to release energy or move muscles.

Water is a polar molecule. One side has a positive charge and the other side has a negative charge, like a magnet or a battery. Like a magnet, the positively charged side of the water will attract the negatively charged molecules, and the negative side will attract positively charged molecules. Like a battery, the concentration of negative and positive ions on either side of water can create a flow of electrons and create energy.

Another type of movement that water is necessary for is diffusion. Chemicals will flow from an area of high concentration to an area of low concentration. For instance, put a drop of food coloring in a cup of water. It doesn't just remain a droplet surrounded by water; it spreads out through the water until each chemical food coloring molecule is evenly distributed.

This type of reaction happens constantly in our

bodies. When our cells deplete certain chemicals that they need to make energy, they need more of those same chemicals to enter the cell. But if the cell, which is mostly made up of water, is dehydrated, then the concentration levels will be off.

If you dropped the food coloring into a half a cup of water, the solution would be darker than if you dropped the same amount in a cup of water. Even though it is the same amount of food coloring, the concentration is higher (and darker) in less water. The same concept is true for the color of your urine. Darker urine means you have less water in your system, which is why urine color is a valid indicator of whether you are well hydrated or not.

When you are even slightly dehydrated, the concentrations of important chemicals in your body can be modified, causing the body to be inefficient at important processes including producing the energy you need to get through your day.

Finally, the third vital function of water is to provide the coolant your body uses to maintain optimal temperature. Your body works best and produces the maximum amount of energy when it is in homeostasis, which means all the systems are running properly. The body's processes are designed to work optimally at around 98.7°F. Water keeps the body's temperature stable, but when you are dehydrated, your body temperature can rise too quickly.

Sweat is the most noticeable use of water to keep your body cool. But water also insulates the inside of your body. When chemical reactions in the body produce heat, water helps absorb that heat so it doesn't spread to nearby structures and cause damage. If body heat rises above about 100.5°F, which is called hyperthermia or a fever, energy production is compromised.

As you can see, even just slight dehydration can cause a lack of energy and increased feelings of tiredness.

How much water should I drink?

Drinking enough water is vital for supercharging your energy levels. Yet scientists estimate that 60 to 90 percent of us are dehydrated daily. There are two reasons for this; we don't know how much we are supposed to drink, and we can't rely on our body's cues to get enough.

The typically recommended eight 8-ounce glasses of water a day is a simple calculation based on the estimated water loss through normal body functions like sweating and breathing. For a person lying in bed all day, 64 ounces may be all you need to keep your body hydrated. Patients in the hospital who require fluid restrictions are still given a minimum of two liters of fluid, a little over 67 ounces. Unless you are bedridden, you are going to need a lot more than eight 8-ounce glasses of water a day.

This will also depend on your size. A smaller person will need less water, a larger person will need more. Exercising or increased activity will increase your need for water. Factors such as diet and overall health will also impact the amount of water you should drink.

Because this isn't complicated enough, there is no one single answer for what a person should drink, and it can vary from day to day for even the same person. So how do we know we are drinking enough?

A good starting point that experts are now using is to drink one half your body weight in ounces of water. If you weigh 160 lbs, you should start by drinking 80 oz of water a day. Then you can use your urine as a gauge. Evaluating your urine color will help you understand how your body uses water during your activities. Urine should be very pale yellow. If it is dark at all, you need more water.

It is not easy in our busy, fast-paced world to drink the amount of water we need, which is why a majority of us are constantly dehydrated. Drinking water has to be a habit in order for our bodies to get enough of it.

"Drink when thirsty" doesn't work for most of us. We tend to ignore our body's signals or reach for beverages other than water when we feel thirst: sodas, coffee, tea, juices, sports drinks, the list goes on. Unfortunately, these beverages do not hydrate us, and they are usually laden with sugar or other stimulants. While these drinks may have their place in our culture, they should not be used as a substitute for the water you need on a daily basis.

When your body is well hydrated, it is a well-oiled machine. It is important to note that enough water will give you the energy you need, and if you are feeling sluggish, you should drink more than you already are. If you know you are well hydrated, however, then more water is not necessarily better. It is possible to get water intoxication from drinking too much, and there have been documented deaths from drinking too much water.

This does take a whole lot of water, though. The first case I ever heard about was a water drinking contest. The poor mom was drinking a ton of water to earn her kid a Wii (the contest was Wee for Wii). She won concert tickets, but her family lost in a big way.

The other way water is harmful is if you are not replacing your electrolytes. As in the case of food coloring in water, the more water, the more diluted the food coloring will be. If there is too much water and not enough vitamins and minerals to keep the body functioning properly, it can cause problems.

Again, these instances of water overloading are few and far between and don't happen during normal day to day activity. In my experience, most people are not drinking enough water because either it's not a habit or they're drinking too many other beverages instead. For most of us, drinking an extra glass of water or two during the day is just what we need to banish that energy slump.

You may have heard or read this before and brushed it off as being too simple of a solution. However, knowing the science behind it now, there's no denying that water can keep you feeling energized, motivated, and satisfied. Bonus: it can help you avoid the next energy-sucker: overeating.

6
OVEREATING

"...We are an overfed and undernourished nation digging an early grave with our teeth..."
—Ezra Taft Benson

The first time I heard the phrase "overfed and undernourished," my stomach dropped. This remains the most accurate statement about the standard American diet I have ever come across. We are eating plenty of protein, fat, and carbohydrates to supply the calories we need, but we are missing out on important micronutrients and energy. We are living longer as a species, but we are sicker than ever. It is way too easy to eat too many calories, and studies have shown that eating less calories may enhance the body's ability to fight disease and slow aging.

While it will be interesting to see where future research leads us on the calorie restriction front, we at least know we can gain more energy on a daily basis by avoiding overeating. There are two different types of overeating that will suck your energy. The first is eating a huge meal all at once, like Thanksgiving dinner. The second is the chronic overeating that most people in developed countries are used to.

The stomach can comfortably hold a little over 32 ounces of food and beverage. When you overeat, it can stretch two or three times more. The immediate uncomfortable feeling after you eat too much is your stomach stretching and pushing against other organs. This includes the lungs, so when you eat too much, you can't breathe as deeply. Your oxygen level drops, slowing down your metabolism and digestion, which prolongs the uncomfortable feeling.

Shallow breathing also causes you to feel tired after a large meal. Digestion already takes a lot of energy and blood flow. Then when you slow your system down further by not breathing deeply, your body devotes all its energy to the digestive system and the brain takes a nap. As we lie there in a food coma watching football, our stomach pumps out more and more acid to try to break down all that food.

Enter the dreaded heartburn. Acid builds up, and some of it splashes into the esophagus, causing the burning feeling right in the middle of the chest.

When food enters your intestines, your body sends signals to your brain that you are full. If the food keeps coming though, the overload of these signals can cause nausea.

This feeling lasts the rest of the day as your body attempts to process this huge meal. It is a no-brainer how overeating in this way monopolizes your energy—a literal no-brainer, in fact.

Chronic overeating, however, doesn't cause obvious, immediate discomfort like binge eating does. Chronic overeating is consuming more calories than your body can use on a regular basis. Particularly when eating processed foods, eating a calorie dense diet causes all kinds of energy drain. First, you are spending more energy digesting food than you really need to be. Second, any calories that the body cannot use in the short term are converted to long term storage: fat. Excess fat storage causes hormonal changes in your body that alter the way your mind and body work and has a huge impact on energy levels.

There is real, sound science behind the calories in versus calories out model that most diets are based on. When there is a balance of energy consumed and used, the body can maintain homeostasis easier. The entire body runs more efficiently, and energy levels can be maximized.

But the number of calories alone cannot boost your energy. The quality of your calories matters, too. Eating 1200 calories of chocolate in a day where you burn 1500 calories will not help you maintain energy or lose weight, for that matter. The type of food you consume can positively or negatively affect the way your body functions and the degree of your energy level.

Eating whole foods like fruits and vegetables helps your body feel more satisfied with less calories. Eating processed foods leaves you craving more processed foods without feeling satisfied. The result is such an overabundance of calories and chemicals that the body spends more energy fueling your digestion rather than receiving usable energy to fuel your activity.

It's about time you understand calories

A calorie is a unit of energy, specifically the amount of energy it takes to raise the temperature of one kilogram of water by one degree Celsius. Anything that produces energy can be measured in calories. Gasoline in a car provides the fuel for combustion, which produces heat and can raise the temperature of water. In the scientific sense, gasoline can be measured in calories. Our bodies cannot use gasoline for energy, of course. Our bodies can only use the calories from three sources: carbohydrates, proteins, and fats. This is why food is the human's main fuel source.

Scientists determined how many calories were in specific foods by burning them and measuring how much heat they produced. Scientists then found the number of calories in pure protein, carbohydrate, and fat: four calories per gram of carbohydrate, four calories per gram of protein, and nine calories per gram of fat. Since the number of food sources has grown so much, manufacturers now estimate the number of calories in the foods they make by multiplying the grams of carbohydrate, protein, and fat that are in the food by these base numbers to find the calorie count.

The important thing to remember here is that the calorie count listed on the food label is an estimate of the calories the food has when physically burned—not via literal fire for us, but rather through chemical reactions.

Calories and overeating

While calories are the units we use to estimate the amount of energy a food supplies the body and can be a way to measure overeating, the body is very complex and the types of foods you eat have a bigger impact on superhuman energy than the amount of calories alone. The good news is when you primarily eat a diet that is rich in micronutrients (ie. lots of fruits and vegetables), it is almost impossible to overeat your calories. These nutrient dense foods are also less likely to cause the next energy draining problem: an unhealthy immune response.

7
IMMUNE RESPONSE

"If part of your immune response is always allocated to repairing gut irritation, you are essentially sick all the time."

–Robb Wolf

One of the most important functions of the body is the immune system. It is designed to fix the body when it is broken and get rid of things that don't belong. Unfortunately, the food we eat can cause all kinds of problems within this important system.

Much of the immune system is in the gut—our digestive system. The immune system is given the task of defending us from anything threatening. But what if the food we are eating is the threat itself? That can stimulate the immune system to mobilize and attack either our own digestive systems, other parts of the body, or even cause death as is the case with some severe allergies. In other words, eating foods that are bad for us can sometimes trigger autoimmune disorders—conditions arising from abnormal immune responses in the body that cause the body to turn on itself!

An allergy is an immune response to something in the environment that is not necessarily harmful to everyone. Allergies are specific to an individual, although there are some allergens that affect large numbers of people. For example, peanut allergies are an immune response to peanuts and can be severe. You have also probably heard of gluten allergies or sensitivity, which is a hot button issue right now. Less severe allergies can be common but unknown because the symptoms are hard to define. The easiest way to find out if certain foods trigger an immune response in your body is to get a food allergy test. An elimination diet, like the Whole30, can also help you understand what foods cause inflammation in your body.

While most people will not experience food allergies to whole foods, studies show that processed and chemical laden foods cause the immune system to activate in the body, causing inflammation. Inflammation makes you feel tired in several ways. In the last decade, research has shown that inflammation in the body causes inflammation in the brain. This slows everything down and can cause you to feel tired and fatigued.

Chemicals released by the body during an immune response can make you feel tired by affecting areas of the brain that regulate alertness and tiredness. These chemicals can also decrease serotonin in the brain, which is one of the chemicals that helps keeps you awake and alert during the day.

Even if you do not have a severe food allergy, the food you eat may be causing inflammation in your body either from specific reactions or a general response to eating chemicals from a lab that the body doesn't recognize as food. This inflammation drains your energy.

Nutrition and immunity

Nutrition has long been tied to our immunity, but most of us have only thought of it passively. "Feed a cold, starve a fever," my grandmother used to say. Most of us have heard of taking massive amounts of vitamin C when we're sick. And there's just something soothing about chicken noodle soup when you are under the weather.

The reality is that what we eat on a regular basis determines when and how long we are sick way more than what we consume while we are sick. Our immune systems encounter many, many pathogens—the bacteria, viruses, germs, or however you think of the "bugs" that make us sick—every single day. There are bacteria on our skin. There are bacteria in our food. We have a whole world of bacteria and fungi inside our bodies.

In fact, research has shown that the bacteria in the gut are an important part of a healthy immune system— the type and health of these microbes greatly impacts your overall health.

There is a huge party going on inside your body, but not everyone is invited. Our immune system is like the bouncer for the party. If a certain bacteria strain is not on the list, your immune system will kick it out. It's those persistent buggers that cause a fight. And when the immune system fights, you feel it—with a sore throat, runny nose, fever, fatigue, etc.

When we eat a diet that is lacking nutrients or causing changes in our bodies' functions (such as the high sugar diet we discussed earlier), our bouncers are kind of puny. Wimpy little guys, who can get the job done in numbers, but almost always require backup and make the fight drag on for days.

When we eat a diet that is rich in nutrients and boosts the body's overall function, our bouncers are huge, buff dudes that kick unwanted pathogens out of the body without any interruption. If they're really good at their jobs, we might not even know we ever had the bug. If you have wimpy bouncers, it takes more energy to fight off the germs we encounter every day. Even though you might not be fully "sick," your energy levels can plummet from your immune system simply being activated. Getting the right nutrients will help buff up your bouncers, which will help keep your energy up on a daily basis and keep you healthier.

Similarly to how the right foods enhance your immune system, the wrong foods can agitate your immune system. Inflammation occurs when your immune system is fighting or repairing your body. When you get a cut on your skin, your body goes to work right away to repair it, activating your immune system. The area bleeds, and gets red. It will sometimes get puffy and hot. These are all immune functions, repairing the cut. Even without broken skin, like when you stub your toe—first there is pain, then the poor toe usually gets red and swollen. This is the immune system repairing damage.

If you eat food that causes inflammation in your body, then your digestive tract gets irritated—just like your stubbed toe. It can bleed. It can get red, puffy, and sometimes hot. Only we call it bloated. We sense that we don't feel superb, but since the immune response is out of sight, it's hard to determine that a particular food is the culprit.

What makes it even tougher is that everybody reacts differently to different foods. I'm sure you've heard of gluten—a protein found in wheat that has become a notorious celebrity. Yes, some people have an autoimmune response when gluten gets into their system—due to celiac disease or gluten sensitivity—and it can have severe consequences. But not everyone reacts in this way. If you are not sensitive to gluten, then you will not see any difference in immune response if you eat it or not. Just like eating or not eating peanuts will do nothing if you are not allergic to them.

If you suspect certain foods cause digestive discomfort, you may want to get some food allergy testing done. It is fascinating to discover what your body is reacting to. But if tests aren't your thing, then you can find out for yourself what foods are sucking your energy by listening to your body and tracking what you eat and how it makes you feel.

8
RECIPES FOR ENERGY

"I think of dieting, then I eat pizza."

–Lara Stone

I would be remiss if I didn't arm you with a few recipes to get you started on your way to more energy. While it is not my intention to saddle you with a "diet," I know it is difficult to start eating differently when you've been eating the same things year in and year out.

The following are some of my family's favorite energizing recipes. I hope they inspire you to put into practice what you have learned in this book!

Breakfast

I spent so many years rolling my eyes at clichés like "You are what you eat," and "Breakfast is the most important meal of the day." Yet here I am, spouting them off in my first book. The difference is the scientific proof

I now possess, as we talked about in chapter 1. But I'm not saying that eating a carbohydrate loaded breakfast first thing in the morning is the most important thing you can do. Some people need to eat within an hour of waking, some like to wait several hours. Either is fine. What is important is that when you break your fast, no matter what time it is, you need nutrient dense, high energy fuel.

Energizing Egg Muffins

This delicious breakfast can be as unique as you are. Swap the vegetables in this recipe for the ones you love the most to not only give your body the energy boost you crave, but give your brain a boost as well!

Makes 12 muffins

Ingredients
10 large eggs
1/2 cup diced bell pepper, any color
1/2 cup diced tomato
1/4 cup diced green onion
1 diced jalapeno (optional)

Instructions
1. Preheat oven to 350 degrees. Prepare muffin tin by applying non-stick spray to silicone baking cups.

2. Scramble eggs in a large bowl. Add the rest of the

vegetables to the eggs. Whisk until ingredients are mixed in and eggs are slightly frothy.

3. Add 1/4 cup of egg mixture to each baking cup. Use any leftover mixture to even out the amount in each cup.

4. Bake for 20 - 25 minutes.

5. Serve warm or refrigerate for breakfast or snack another day. My kids will eat these straight from the fridge!

Snacks

Sneaky snack attacks can mean the downfall of your energy for the rest of the day. When we get that need-to-eat-right-this-second feeling, we tend to reach for the most convenient food available with the boldest flavor. Usually this involves something processed straight from a bag. The easiest way to combat this energy sucking habit is to have energizing snacks on hand for those moments!

Energizing Trail Mix

This trail mix will spark your creativity. Substitute the mixed nuts for two or three of your all-time favorite nuts. Swap the goji and/or mulberries with dried cranberries, strawberries, or blueberries. For ultimate energy, cacao nibs (raw, unprocessed chocolate) is rich in micronutrients and antioxidants. Plus, they give a rich flavor to complement the sweetness of the dried berries and the satisfying proteins and fats of the nuts.

Ingredients
2 cups raw, unsalted mixed nuts
1 cup dried goji berries
1 cup dried mulberries
1/2 cup cacao nibs

Instructions
Place all ingredients in an airtight container of choice, mix, and enjoy by the handful! Store in a cool, dry place.

Lunch

Lunch is all too often an afterthought; then we find ourselves at the mercy of our must-eat-now state. Combat the monster by planning ahead. Leftovers of your nutrient rich dinner the night before make an excellent lunch choice. If you ordered pizza last night, though, you'd be better off with a good salad chock full of micronutrient dense vegetables.

Salads can be as basic or ornate as you want them to be. Personally, I prefer spinach and kale, topped with diced tomatoes, cucumber, and thinly sliced onion.

No matter which vegetables (or fruits) you add, the key is the dressing. Healthy fats signal satisfaction to the brain, allowing you to feel full. Low-fat dressings can leave you feeling completely unsatisfied after a salad. Combat this feeling by adding whole foods containing healthy fats, such as nuts or avocados, or using my favorite, super simple homemade dressing!

Satisfying Salad Dressing

This dressing will add satisfaction to your salad with full flavor, satisfying oils, and micronutrient dense herbs!

Makes 1 cup of dressing

Ingredients

3/4 cup olive oil

1/4 cup balsamic vinegar

1/4 teaspoon dried oregano

1/4 teaspoon dried basil

1/8 teaspoon garlic powder

Instructions

Mix all ingredients together in a container. Shake well before serving. Use 1 - 2 tablespoons per serving. Store in a cool, dark place.

Dinner

While on my quest to find flavorful, healthy dinner recipes with nutritious ingredients my family enjoys, I was drawn to the flavor-packed Jambalaya. Each recipe I found, however, used white or brown rice. Quick cooking white or brown rice doesn't pack the wallop of micronutrients that long grain brown rice contains. Long grain brown rice cooks very differently as well. I took to my test kitchen and created this Jambalaya recipe with the extra punch of nutrient dense long grain brown rice. The leftovers make a fantastic lunch the next day as well!

Energizing Jambalaya
Makes 4 Servings

Ingredients
8 ounces chicken, diced
12 oz andouille sausage
1 Tbsp. Creole seasoning
2 Tbsp. olive oil
1/2 cup chopped onion
1/2 cup chopped green bell pepper
1/2 cup chopped celery
2 cloves minced garlic
1/2 cup chopped tomatoes
3 bay leaves
3/4 cup brown rice
3 1/2 cups chicken stock
salt and pepper

Instructions

1. In a large saucepan or pot, heat oil over high heat. Add onion, pepper and celery, stirring occasionally until slightly tender, about 5 minutes. Add garlic, tomatoes, bay leaves, and creole seasoning. Stir for an additional 2 minutes to blend flavors. Stir in rice and broth. Bring to a boil, then reduce heat to medium, cover, and cook until rice absorbs liquid and becomes tender, stirring rarely, about 45 minutes to 1 hour.

2. While rice is cooking, prepare chicken and andouille sausage. Dice sausage and chicken. If pre-cooked, set aside to add to rice. To cook, heat 1 tbsp oil in a pan, and add diced chicken and sausage. Heat, stirring, until cooked through, about 10 minutes.

3. When rice is just tender remove bay leaves then add sausage and chicken mixture. Cook until heated through, about 5 minutes more.

4. Season to taste with salt, pepper and Creole seasoning.

CONCLUSION

Welcome, friend, to the end of the book! Congratulations on reading this far. Your head may be reeling—I pretty much just told you everything you are eating and drinking is draining your energy. But I promise you: you can do it!

Your journey to ultimate energy and the superhuman version of yourself is just beginning! This book contains everything you need to get started. Commit to drinking water instead of soda tomorrow. Choose one of the high energy breakfast recipes in this book and forego your sugary Pop-tarts in the morning. Skip the breakroom donut and snack on some raw, unsalted nuts instead.

You can achieve the superhuman energy you need to give your 100 percent to everything you do . . . one meal at a time!

ABOUT THE AUTHOR

Jadie Aranda is a passionate biologist who secretly teaches people science so they can live better lives. As a scientist and skeptic of all the diet misinformation fed to consumers, Jadie works tirelessly to sift through scientific publications, distill the truth, and share it with her readers in an understandable and engaging way.

When she doesn't have her nose stuck in the latest research, Jadie enjoys life in Colorado with her husband and two amazing children. Visit **www.EatMyScience.com** and **www.JadieAranda.com** for more!

THANK YOU!

I hope you have enjoyed Your High Energy Life! While the book is fresh on your mind, please go to Amazon and leave a review with your honest opinion of the information you just read. I value your feedback greatly, and other readers will benefit from your experience.

Thank you from the bottom of my heart, you fantastic human, you!